Pressing RESET for Respiratory Illness

original strength

Original strength

Pressing Reset for Respiratory Illness
by OS Press

Copyright © 2020 Original Strength Systems, LLC

ALL RIGHTS RESERVED.

All rights reserved solely by the copyright holder. The copyright holder guarantees all contents are original and do not infringe upon the legal rights of any other person or work. No part of this book may be reproduced or transmitted in any form or by any means, electronic or mechanical, including photocopying, recording or by any information storage and retrieval system, without the permission of the copyright holder or the publisher.

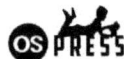

Published by OS Press - Fuquay-Varina, NC

Contributors:

Tim Anderson
Co-Founder, Original Strength Systems

Dani Almeyda, MS
Education Director, Original Strength Institute

Peiting Lien, PT, DPT
Board Certified Specialist in Neurological Physical Therapy,
Johns Hopkins Rehabilitation Network

Ken Johnson, PT
Director of Outpatient Rehabilitation Therapy Services at Johns Hopkins Hospital and physical therapist at Johns Hopkins Rehabilitation Network

Jennifer Zanni, PT, DScPT
Board Certified Specialist in Cardiovascular and Pulmonary Physical Therapy, Johns Hopkins Rehabilitation Network

ISBNs:
Paperback: 978-1-64184-369-0

Thank you to JETLAUNCH.net for editing and book design.

Medical Disclaimer

You must get your physician's approval before beginning this program. These recommendations are not medical guidelines but are for educational purposes only. You must consult your physician prior to starting this program or if you have any medical condition or injury that is contraindicated to performing physical activity.

See your physician before starting any exercise or nutrition program. If you are taking any medications, you must talk to your physician before starting any exercise program. If you experience any lightheadedness, dizziness, or shortness of breath while exercising, stop the movement and consult a physician.

It is strongly recommended that you have a complete physical examination if you live a sedentary lifestyle, have high cholesterol, high blood pressure, diabetes, are overweight, or if you are over thirty years old. Please discuss all nutritional changes with your physician or a registered dietician. Please follow your doctor's orders.

All forms of exercise pose some inherent risks. The contributors—authors, editors, and publishers—advise readers to take full responsibility for their safety and know their limits. When using the exercises in this program, do not move into pain.

Pressing
RESET

Pressing Reset on Respiratory Illness

The Impact

Respiratory illnesses vary in severity and cause. Regardless of their severity, they impact the whole person, and they can have a lasting effect. It should not be dismissed that the stress surrounding a respiratory illness has a great effect on the mind and emotions. This impact can lead to bouts of fear and depression, both of which will further compromise the health of the individual.

As respiratory illnesses attack and affect the whole person (the body, mind, and emotions), recovery efforts should also be aimed at restoring the whole person in order for them to return to their previous and desired quality of life.

The Solution: Pressing Reset on the Whole Person

Movement heals the body, and it can also lead to the healing of the whole person. Movement is the "back door" to restoring the mind and soothing the emotions. Through engaging in specific movements that are preprogrammed inside every person's nervous system, we can begin the process of restoration and healing.

The body is designed to heal and repair itself through movement. There are Three Pillars of Human Movement that repair and optimize the whole person's health in body, mind, and emotions.

They are:

1. **Breathe deep with the diaphragm** - belly breathe, filling the lungs up from the bottom to the top
2. **Activate the vestibular system** - this is the balance and sensory integration system of the body
3. **Cross midline** or engage in contralateral patterns like crawling, marching, or walking

These three pillars are preprogrammed into every individual's nervous system, and they are woven into the developmental sequence. The purpose of the developmental sequence is to build and strengthen the nervous system as well as strengthen the body. These movements remain inside the nervous system throughout a person's life, regardless of their age.

If the three pillars of human movement, or the developmental movements, are engaged in, they will do what they were designed to do: build and strengthen the nervous system, strengthening the entire person: body, mind, and emotions. This is the original design of the whole body—to repair and recover throughout life. We call this design your original strength.

Your body is awesomely and wonderfully made. Living in your design, moving with your original strength allows you to live your life better, the way you want to. It gives you the freedom to move and the ability to enjoy your life. This original strength lives inside of you, and it is released when you move according to your design.

The Method: Pressing RESET

The following movements are targeted at one purpose: to help the patient return to their way of life and enjoy full health. They will be presented in different stages of recovery and should be engaged in according to the severity of the patient's condition. In other words, each patient should "Start where they are."

Precautions

Do not begin exercises if:

- You have a fever
- You have any shortness of breath or difficulty breathing
- You have any chest pain or palpitations ("fluttering" of heart in the chest)
- You have any new swelling in your legs

STOP the exercises immediately if you develop any of the following symptoms:

- Dizziness
- Shortness of breath
- Chest pain
- Cool, clammy skin
- Excessive fatigue
- Palpitations

Seek help immediately for chest pain, shortness of breath that does not resolve with rest, and dizziness that does not resolve with rest or any change in mental status from baseline.

RECOVERY STAGE: SEVERE

IF YOU ARE RECOVERING FROM A SEVERE RESPIRATORY ILLNESS AND YOU HAVE TO REMAIN IN BED FOR MOST OF THE DAY, START HERE.

Reset #1

Severe Recovery Stage: Breath Focus

This stage is suitable for patients recovering from a severe respiratory illness, resulting in an ICU visit (intubation, mechanical breathing assistance, bedridden for a prolonged period, ARDS). *Patients in this stage would be recovering in a bed and may or may not have the strength to sit unassisted.*

If you are recovering from a severe respiratory illness and you have to remain in bed for most of the day, start here.

These exercises may be initiated even if you still feel very weak and are lying down for the majority of the day. Your breathing should feel unlabored at rest, and you should be able to comfortably speak in full sentences while performing these exercises.

Movement #1

Breathing

This is where we are going to start. We are aiming to restore diaphragmatic and lung function. This is also where the restoration of mind and emotions begins, as well as breathing, which is the bridge between Panic Mode (sympathetic nervous system) and Restoration Mode (parasympathetic nervous system).

YAWN TO A SMILE

Yawning relieves tension in the muscles of the face. The nerves of the face are neurologically connected to the diaphragm. Relieving tension in the face relieves stress and tension throughout the entire body, and it allows the diaphragm to function more easily. Smiling also relieves tension in the face, but it also causes the release of "feel good" endorphins and actually reduces the perception of pain.

- Lie on your back in a comfortable position.
- Create a big yawn and finish it by smiling for three seconds.
- Do this three times.

DIAPHRAGMATIC BREATHING (BELLY BREATHING)

Diaphragmatic breathing restores the function of the diaphragm and fills the lungs up from the bottom to the top. Breathing through the nose strengthens the diaphragm and encourages the nervous system to operate in Restoration Mode.

- Lie on your back, bend your knees so that the bottom of your feet are resting on your bed.
- Place your hands on top of your belly or wrap them around the sides of your belly.
- Close your lips and place your tongue on the roof of your mouth.
- Breathe in through your nose and pull air down into your belly where your hands are. Try to lift your hands up and down or spread your fingers apart with your breath.
- Do this for one minute.

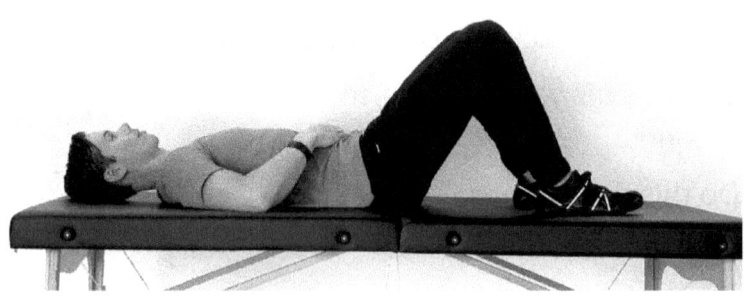

PURSED LIP EXHALATION (SLOWLY BLOWING OUT A CANDLE)

Exhaling with pursed lips creates more intra-abdominal pressure; thus, it helps to stabilize the core. This extra pressure also creates the opportunity for the diaphragm to have a stronger reflexive rebound on inhalation. Exhaling slowly with pursed lips also increases exhalation time, soothing the nervous system and relieving stress (Restoration Mode).

- Lie on your back with knees bent or with legs straight.
- Place your hands on top of your belly or wrap them around the sides of your belly.
- With your lips closed and your tongue on the roof of your mouth, breathe in through your nose and pull air down into your belly where your hands are. Try to lift your hands or spread your fingers apart with your breath.
- Once your lungs are full, pierce your lips and slowly let the air out of your lungs. Notice how your hands lower back down.
- Inhale through your nose, exhale through pursed lips.
- Do this for one minute.

HUMMING

Humming while exhaling helps increase nitric oxide production in the body. Nitric oxide helps with neural plasticity (helps the nervous system build and repair) and dilates blood vessels, enabling more oxygen to be delivered throughout the body. Humming is also calming and soothing; it reduces stress and can help one remain in Restoration Mode.

- Lie on your back with knees bent or with legs straight.
- Place your hands on top of your belly or wrap them around the sides of your belly.
- With your lips closed and your tongue on the roof of your mouth, breathe in through your nose and pull air down into your belly where your hands are. Try to lift your hands or spread your fingers apart with your breath.
- Once your lungs are full, keep your lips close and exhale while humming. Make the "hmmmmmm" sound. Notice how your hands lower back down.
- Inhale through your nose, exhale through your nose while humming.
- Do this for one minute.

Movement #2
Activating the Vestibular System

The Vestibular System is the system that establishes balance, posture, and coordination. It is also the crossroads of all information received and generated by the body. Activating the vestibular system improves the strength of the body and helps balance emotions.

EYE NODS

Nodding the eyes up and down stimulates the vestibular system and restores reflexive muscular connections throughout the body. When paired with breathing, eye nods can be used to develop coordination in timing, strengthening neural connections in the brain while providing additional focus on the breath.

- Sit up in your bed in a comfortable position.
- Close your lips and place your tongue on the roof of your mouth.
- Look up with your eyes and breathe in through your nose. Try to pull air down into your belly.
- As you exhale through your nose, look down with your eyes.
- Try to hold your eyes up as you inhale and down as you exhale.
    - » This should be a relaxed, easy breath, so it is slow.

- Move the eyes up and down as far as they will comfortably move.
- Do this for one minute.

BED ROLLING

Rolling from side to side further activates the vestibular system and also integrates the sensory systems (visual, vestibular, proprioceptive). It provides the body with a good "movement map." When paired with breathing, rolling can also help teach relaxation and can be a great way to relieve stress while strengthening the body.

- Lie on your back in a comfortable position.
- Look to the right with your eyes.
- Rotate your head to the right.
- Roll your body to the right so that you are on your side.
- Take a deliberate breath or two.
- Then, look to the left with your eyes.
- Rotate your head to the left.
- Roll your body to the left until you end up on your left side.
- Take a deliberate breath or two before rolling to the right again.
- First the eyes, then the head, then the body.
- Roll from side to side at a relaxed pace for 2 minutes.

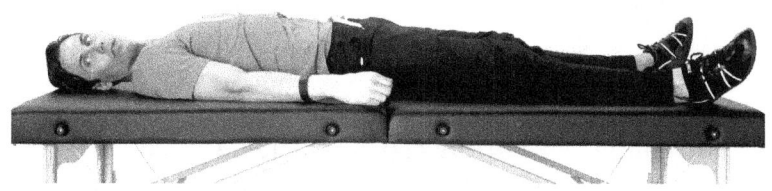

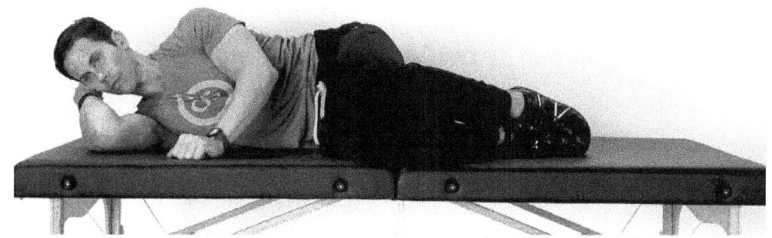

Movement #3

Crossing Midline

Crossing midline is simply crossing the centerline of your body with your arms or legs. Crossing the centerline of the body increases the communication between the two hemispheres of the brain. It makes the brain more efficient at communicating with the rest of the body, allowing the body to move better with more strength and stability. Crossing midline also improves cognitive function, memory, and focus.

CROSS-CRAWL TOUCHES

- Lie on your back in a comfortable position.
- Take your right hand and touch your left thigh. If you are able, you can lift your left leg to meet your right hand.
- Then take your left hand and touch your right thigh. If you are able, you can lift your right leg to meet your left hand.
- Work these touches from side to side for one minute.

If you are in this stage, work through this routine two times per day.

RECOVERY STAGE:
MILD

IF YOU ARE RECOVERING FROM A MILD RESPIRATORY ILLNESS, OR IF YOU ARE NOW STRONG ENOUGH TO SIT UNASSISTED AND UPRIGHT, AND YOU HAVE STRENGTH TO NAVIGATE THROUGH YOUR HOME FOR SHORT PERIODS OF TIME, START HERE.

Reset #2

Mild Recovery Stage: Vestibular System Focus

This stage is suitable for patients recovering from a mild respiratory illness—suffering from more mild cases, which could include hospitalization (minimal hospitalization and sent home to self-isolate while they recover). *Patients in this stage would be able to sit unassisted and may be able to navigate through their homes for short durations.*

If you are recovering from a mild respiratory illness, or if you are now strong enough to sit unassisted and upright, and you have the strength to navigate through your home for short periods of time, start now.

Movement #1
Breathing

YAWN TO A SMILE

- Sit upright on the edge of your bed or in a sturdy chair.
- Reach your arms overhead and create a big stretching yawn and finish it by smiling for three seconds.
- Do this three times.

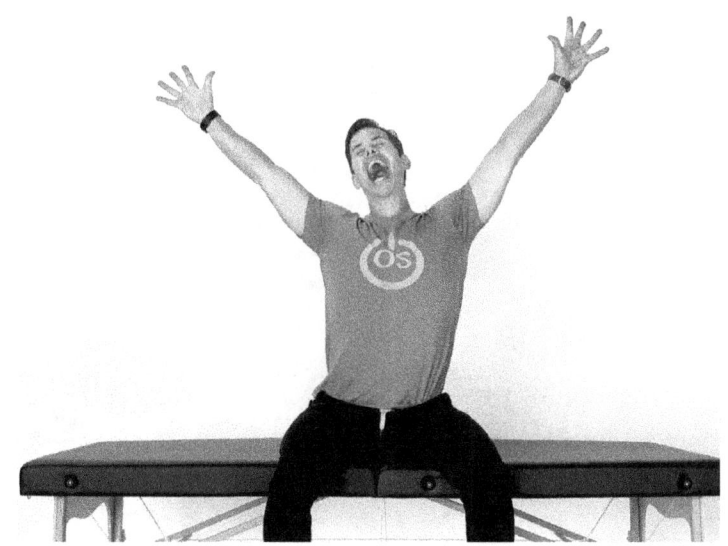

DIAPHRAGMATIC BREATHING (BELLY BREATHING)

- Sit upright on the edge of your bed or in a sturdy chair.
- Place your hands around the sides of your belly.
- Close your lips and place your tongue on the roof of your mouth.
- Breathe in through your nose and pull air down into your belly where your hands are. Try to spread your fingers apart with your breath.
- Do this for one minute.

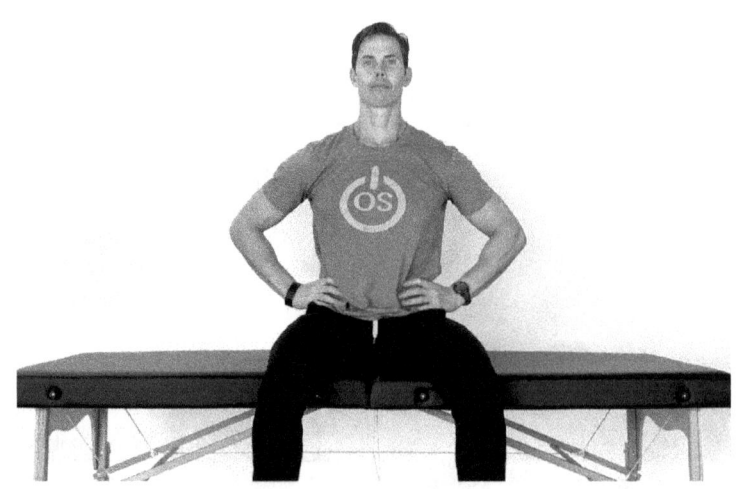

PURSED LIP EXHALATION (SLOWLY BLOWING OUT A CANDLE)

- Stand upright as tall as you can and place your hands around your waist.
- Place your hands around the sides of your belly.
- With your lips closed and your tongue on the roof of your mouth,
- breathe in through your nose and pull air down into your belly where your hands are. Try to spread your fingers apart with your breath.
- Once your lungs are full, purse your lips and slowly let the air out of your lungs.
- Inhale through your nose, exhale through pursed lips.
- Do this for one minute.

Movement #2

Activating the Vestibular System

HEAD NODS

Head nods are the continuation of eyes nods performed in Phase 1. Head nods reflexively engage the core and postural muscles, strengthening the body from the center.

Sit upright on the edge of your bed or in a sturdy chair.

- Close your lips and place your tongue on the roof of your mouth.
- Inhale through your nose and look up with your eyes and then lift your head as far as you comfortably can.
- As you exhale through your nose, look down with your eyes and lower your chin towards your chest.
- Try to match the movement of your eyes and head to the rhythm of your breath, nodding your head up as you inhale and lowering your head down as you exhale.
    - » This should be a relaxed, easy breath, so it is slow.
- Move the eyes and head up and down as far as they will comfortably move.
- Do this for one minute.

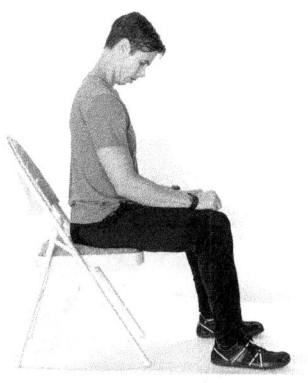 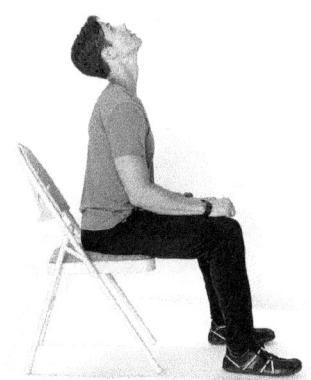

HEAD ROTATIONS

Like head nods, head rotations reflexively engage the core and postural muscles. Head rotations also introduce gentle rotation into the cervical and thoracic spine.

- Sit upright on the edge of your bed or in a sturdy chair.
- Close your lips and place your tongue on the roof of your mouth.
- Look to the right with your eyes and rotate your head to the right as if to look behind your right shoulder.
- Then look to the left with your eyes and rotate your head to the left as if to look behind your left shoulder.
- Rotate your head as far as your neck will comfortably allow.
- Do not move into pain.
- Rotate from side to side, as if looking back over your shoulders.
- Do this for one minute.

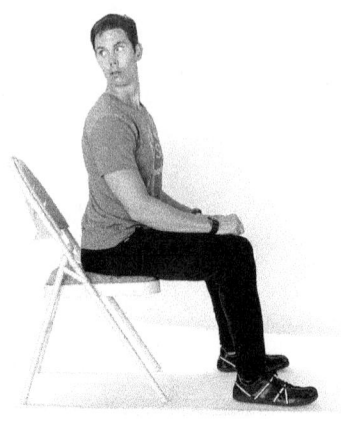 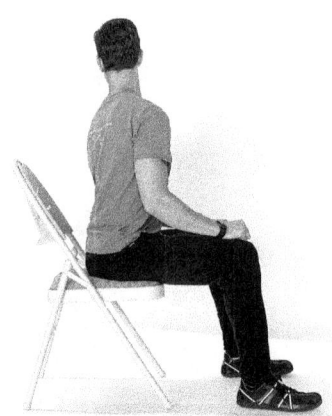

ROCKING

Rocking back and forth while sitting in a chair greatly activates the vestibular system and creates a strong, reflexive relationship between the core muscles of the trunk and the muscles of the neck. Rocking also calms and soothes the emotions. It can help a person enter Restoration Mode or bring them out of Panic Mode, the sympathetic nervous system.

- Sit upright on the edge of your bed or in a sturdy chair.
- Fix your gaze on an object directly in front and level with your eyes.
- Keeping your gaze fixed on an object and your head level with the horizon, inhale and lean back in your chair.
- Then exhale and lean forward towards the object.

- You are essentially rocking back and forth underneath your head while your eyes stay fixed on an object straight in front of you.
- Inhale as you lean back, exhale as your rock forward.
- Do this at a relaxed pace for one minute.

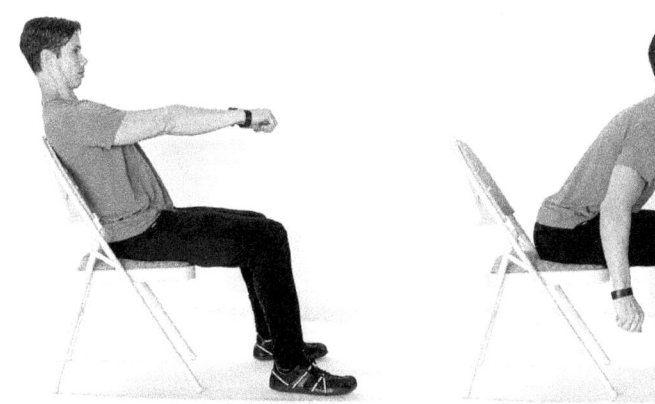

ROCKING TO STAND

Here, we are taking advantage of the reflexive relationship between the core muscles and the neck, and using their momentum to stand. This develops overall coordination in the body as it strengthens the legs.

- Sit upright on the edge of your bed or in a sturdy chair.
- Fix your gaze on an object directly in front and level with your eyes.
- Keeping your gaze fixed on an object and your head level with the horizon, inhale and lean back in your chair.

- Then exhale and lean forward and stand up.
- Sit back down.
- Inhale, lean back.
- Exhale, lean forward, and stand.
- Repeat this at a relaxed pace for one minute.

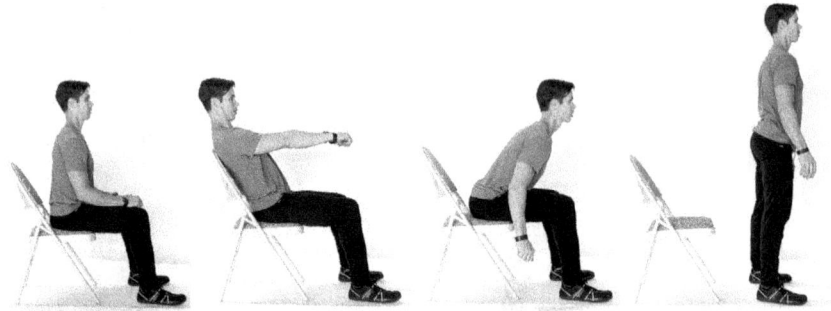

Movement #3
Crossing Midline

SEATED CROSS-CRAWL TOUCHES

- Sit upright on the edge of your bed or in a sturdy chair.
- Reach your arms up overhead.
- Take your right hand and touch your left thigh.
  » If you are able, lift your left thigh to meet your right hand.
- Release the touch and return your right hand overhead.
- Take your left hand and touch your right thigh.
  » If you are able, lift your right thigh to meet your left hand.
- Release the touch and return your left hand overhead.
- Work these touches back and forth, from side to side.
- Do this for one minute at a relaxed pace.

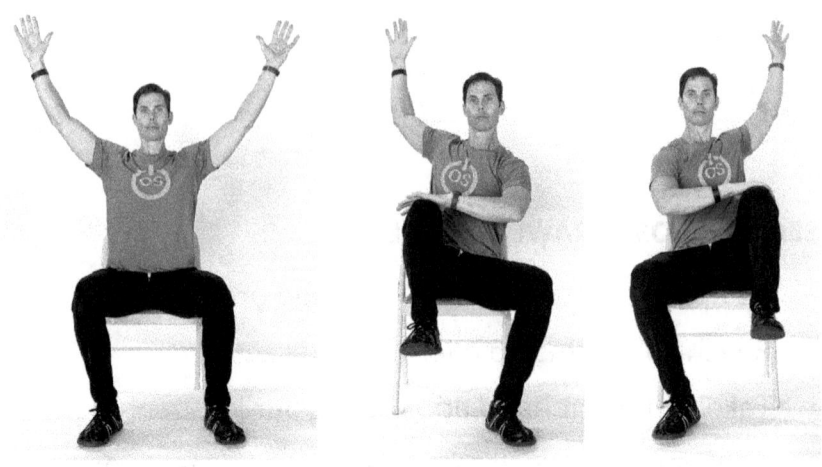

*If you are in this stage, work through this routine two times per day, and **if you can**, take a five- to ten-minute walk while maintaining nasal breathing.*

RECOVERY STAGE: STRENGTH BUILDING

IF YOU CAN GET UP AND DOWN FROM THE FLOOR, AND YOU CAN EASILY NAVIGATE THROUGH YOUR HOME, START HERE.

Reset #3

Strength Recovery Stage: Contralateral Pattern Focus

In this stage, the patient has the strength to get up and down from the floor, they can easily navigate through their home, and they are preparing to resume their way of living before contracting the virus.

If you can get up and down from the floor, and you can easily navigate through your home, start here.

Movement #1
Breathing

YAWN TO A SMILE

- Stand upright with a long spine.
- Reach your arms overhead and create a big stretching yawn and finish it by smiling for three seconds.
- Do this three times.

DIAPHRAGMATIC BREATHING (BELLY BREATHING)

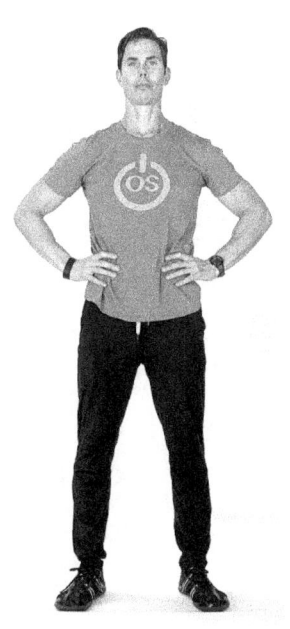

- Stand upright and place your hands around the sides of your belly.
- Close your lips and place your tongue on the roof of your mouth.
- Breathe in through your nose and pull air down into your belly where your hands are. Try to spread your fingers apart with your breath.
- Do this for two minutes.
  - » *You may practice pierced lip exhalation or humming exhalation here if desired.*

Movement #2

Activating the Vestibular System

WINDSHIELD WIPERS

Windshield wipers are a form of rolling. They create gentle rotation in the thoracic and cervical spine. This motion opens the ribcage and frees up shoulder mobility.

- Lie on your back and place your arms perpendicular to your body.
- Close your lips and place your tongue on the roof of your mouth and breathe through your nose.
- Bend your knees and pull your knees up towards your chest (your feet will be in the air).
- Look to the right with your eyes and head and then rotate your legs over to the right.
    - » Try to keep your shoulder blades on the floor.
- Look back to the left with your eyes and your head and then rotate your legs over to the left.
- Keep your knees pulled up towards your chest as you rotate your legs over.
- Work this motion from side to side at a relaxed pace for one minute.

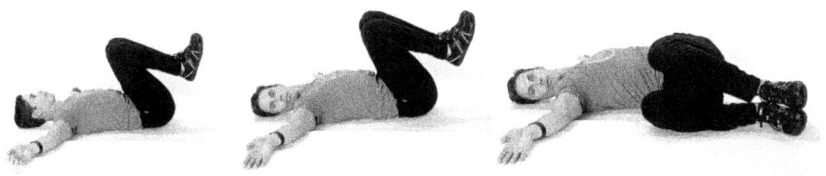

ROCKING ON HANDS AND KNEES

Rocking back and forth on the hands and knees activates the vestibular system and restores the reflexive posture of the spine. Rocking on the hands and knees integrates all the major moving joints of the body through coordinating rhythmic movement. Rocking also soothes the emotions and helps one enter Restoration Mode.

- Get on your hands and knees (this can be done on a bed).
- Hold your head up and fix your gaze on the horizon.
- Close your lips, place your tongue on the roof of your mouth, and breathe through your nose.
- While keeping a "proud chest," rock back towards your feet.
  - » Rock back as far as you comfortably can without dropping your head or rounding your back.

- Then rock forward until your weight is back over your hands.
- Rock back and forth at a relaxed pace for two minutes.

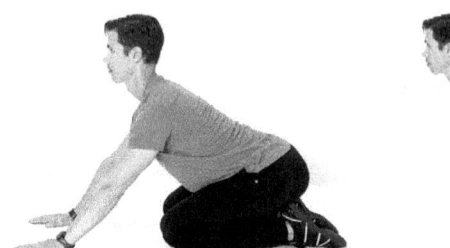 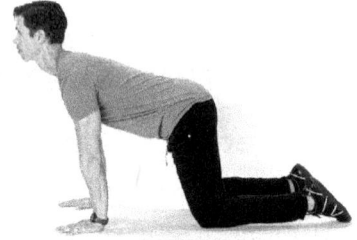

Movement #3

Crossing Midline and Contralateral Patterns

BIRDDOGS

Performing birddogs is a contralateral pattern; it coordinates the opposing limbs to move together. Contralateral patterns strengthen the entire nervous system, but they also tie the body together by creating a reflexively strong center. Birddogs do this by challenging the stability of the body, strengthening the body, and improving balance.

- Get on your hands and knees (this can be done on a bed).
- Hold your head up and fix your gaze on the horizon.
- Close your lips, place your tongue on the roof of your mouth, and breathe through your nose.
- While keeping a "proud chest," lift your right arm and your left leg up and apart from each other. Then lower them down together.
- Then lift your left arm and your right leg up and apart from each other. Then lower them down together.
- Work this back and forth from side to side at a relaxed pace for one minute.

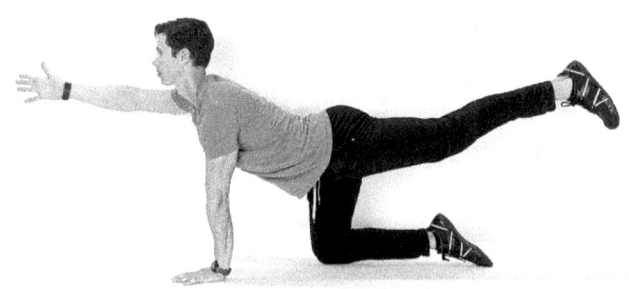

STANDING CROSS-CRAWL TOUCHES

- Stand up "nice and tall."
- Close your lips, place your tongue on the roof of your mouth, and breathe through your nose.
- Touch your opposite limbs together by touching your right hand to your left thigh and your left hand to your right thigh.
  - » If you have the mobility, touch your right elbow to your left knee and your left elbow to your right knee.
- Work this slowly from side to side, touching opposite limbs together for one minute.

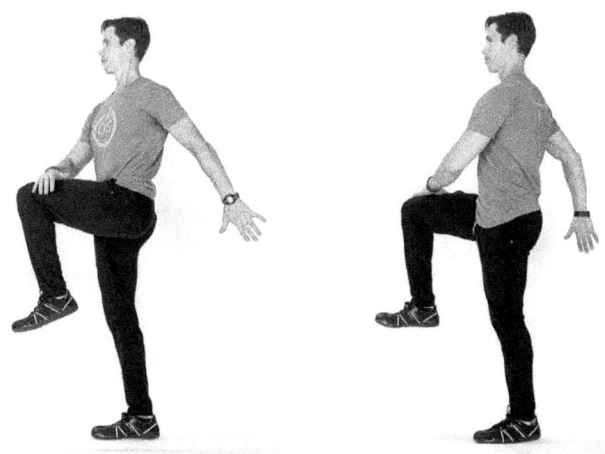

*If you are in this stage, work through this routine two times per day, and **if you can**, take a fifteen- to twenty-minute walk while maintaining nasal breathing.*

From the first to the last - each breath makes a difference

Your body was designed just for you, and Pressing RESET is about working with that design. Your body is built on the three pillars of human movement. When you regularly engage in these three things, your body will try to work the way it was designed to work. Your nervous system will begin sending out messages throughout your body to help you build from where you are at.

Recovery can begin with a simple smile to a yawn or relearning how to breathe with your diaphragm - even humming can get your body on the path to recovery. You can further your recovery and continue rebuilding yourself by adding in eye nods, and rolling in bed, and performing some simple cross-lateral movements. Finally, when you are able, engaging in the strength-building stage will further enhance your recovery and allow you to enjoy your body's amazing design.

You may have started out with a respiratory issue, but remember your whole body, mind, and emotions are affected by illness. These movements will help you recover, and they will strengthen all of You. As you Press RESET, you may notice improvements quickly, or they may take time, just be patient, and keep doing them.

You can grow stronger. You can feel better. Know that. Move within your design with that knowledge. Remember how to smile, how to breathe, how to move your head, how to move your limbs. Remember that you are wonderfully made and live your best life. Keep us informed at PressingRESETfor@originalstrength.net

Want to Learn More?

Original Strength is an education company that teaches about the power of human movement and how it can change the world.

This booklet was designed to give you a brief overview of some of the RESETS we do in Original Strength and apply them to your recovery from respiratory illness. Along the way, you may begin to notice that you feel and move better in general. Feel free to feel good as much as you'd like!

We put this together because we know Pressing RESET can help everyone and anyone. If you do nothing more than what is in this booklet, you will notice many changes in how your body moves and feels. It will benefit both your mind and body.

At Original Strength, we teach health, fitness, and education professionals how to get more out of their patients, clients, athletes, and students. The Original Strength System will reestablish a foundation of movement that will make any physical goal easier and more attainable and help improve mental acuity. We do this by conducting clinics, courses, and training designed for professionals in the fitness, health, wellness, sports conditioning, and vestibular and neuromuscular functionality sectors.

If you want to know more about Pressing RESET and regaining your original strength, visit www.originalstrength.net. There you will find a variety of books, free video tutorials (Movement Snax), and a complete listing of our courses, clinics, and OS Certified Professionals near you.

You may want to consider finding an OS Certified Professional. These professionals can conduct an Original Strength Screen and Assessment (OSSA), which is the quickest and easiest way to identify areas your movement system needs to go from good to best. The OSSA allows your OS Professional to pinpoint the best place for you to start Pressing RESET and restoring your original strength.

If you want to feel good and live life better and stronger, find an OS Certified Professional near you.

Press RESET now and live life better
because you were awesomely and
wonderfully made to accomplish
amazing things.

For more information:

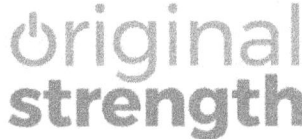

Original Strength Systems, LLC
OriginalStrength.net

PressingRESETfor@Originalstrength.net

"... I am fearfully and wonderfully made..."
Psalm 139:14

www.ingramcontent.com/pod-product-compliance
Lightning Source LLC
Chambersburg PA
CBHW071127030426
42336CB00013BA/2226